RAND Health

Managed Care

Evaluation and Adoption of

Emerging Medical Technologies

Executive Summary

Steven Garber ◆ M. Susan Ridgely ◆ Roger S. Taylor ◆ Robin Meili

Supported by the Health Industry Manufacturers Association,
the California Goldstrike Partnership, and the U.S. Economic Development Administration

RAND

New medical technologies—pharmaceuticals, medical devices, and procedures—often allow great improvements in the outcomes of medical care, but they are also widely believed to be a major cause of increasing costs. Selective adoption of new technologies, the taking on of only those technologies for which the medical benefits exceed the costs to society of developing and using them, is a crucial element in the quest to control health care costs while preserving or enhancing the quality of care.

This document summarizes a project examining adoption of innovative medical technologies by managed care organizations (MCOs). The project had two primary objectives: (1) to understand how MCOs make coverage, medical-necessity, and payment decisions involving emerging medical technologies, and how device developers and manufacturers prepare for and participate in these processes; and (2) to identify ways that private, voluntary action by the managed-care and medical-device industries might improve—for the benefit of society—the processes by which new medical technologies are developed, evaluated, and adopted or rejected for coverage.

The analysis is based on information from in-depth, semi-structured interviews with eight manufacturers of innovative devices and nine managed care organizations and on literature bearing on issues raised by the interviews. The research team also collected information from representatives of manufacturers, MCOs, and the study sponsors—the California Goldstrike Partnership, the Economic Development Administration of the U.S. Department of Commerce, and the Health Industry Manufacturers Association (HIMA)—at a half-day, invitation-only meeting held at RAND headquarters on October 7, 1999. A major contribution of the study is the juxtaposition of manufacturers' reported experiences and perspectives of MCOs.

This executive summary will be of interest to medical-device developers and manufacturers, managed care organizations, public-policy makers, and researchers and analysts. Complete study findings are reported in Steven Garber, M. Susan Ridgely, Roger S. Taylor, and Robin Meili, *Managed Care and the Evaluation and Adoption of Emerging Medical Technologies*, MR-1195-HIMA, RAND, 2000.

This executive summary is based on research conducted under the auspices of RAND Health. RAND Health furthers RAND's mission of helping improve policy and decisionmaking through research and analysis, by working to improve health care systems and advance understanding of how the organization and financing of care affect costs, quality, and access.

CONTENTS

New medical technologies—pharmaceuticals, medical devices, and procedures—often allow major improvements in the outcomes of medical care, but they are also widely believed to be a leading cause of increasing costs. Selective adoption of new technologies, the taking on of only those technologies for which the medical benefits exceed the costs to society of developing and using them, is a crucial element in the quest to control health care costs while preserving or enhancing the quality of care.

The report summarized here focuses on adoption of innovative medical technologies by managed care organizations (MCOs). The project had two primary objectives: (1) to understand current processes of MCOs for making coverage, medical-necessity, and payment decisions involving emerging medical technologies, and how device developers and manufacturers prepare for and participate in these processes; and (2) to identify ways that private, voluntary action by the managed-care and device industries individually or jointly might improve—for the benefit of society—the processes by which new medical technologies are developed, evaluated, and adopted or rejected for coverage.

Extensive information about MCO processes was collected through confidential, in-depth interviews with eight manufacturers of innovative medical devices and medical directors of nine California MCOs, five of which are affiliated with national MCOs. The preliminary findings from these interviews were presented at a meeting on October 7, 1999, at which representatives of manufacturers, MCOs, and the sponsoring organizations—the State of California's

Goldstrike Partnership, the Economic Development Administration of the U.S. Department of Commerce, and the Health Industry Manufacturers Association—critiqued and elaborated on our findings and interpretations. The study is especially novel in collecting and synthesizing information about the experiences and perspectives of manufacturers, and in juxtaposing their reported experiences and perspectives with those of MCOs.

PERSPECTIVES OF MANUFACTURERS

We sought to interview individuals at companies that are actively marketing medical devices that might offer significant medical advances over alternatives but that also might increase costs to MCOs. Each interview addressed four sets of issues:

- Background on the company and the one or two devices on which the interview focused

- The experience of the company in marketing the device or devices to MCOs

- Factors other than MCO behavior affecting adoption of the technology

- Lessons learned and advice for somewhat inexperienced device developers and manufacturers.

Part of the second goal of the project was to develop information that could help manufacturers understand the market environment and to prepare accordingly. Almost all of the interview subjects emphasized early development of commercialization strategies and planning for commercialization efforts. Virtually all manufacturers emphasized that, well before a product is ready for Food and Drug Administration (FDA) review, companies should analyze various issues, including the following:

- Prevalence, incidence, and patient demographics of the disease or medical condition at which the product is aimed

- Effectiveness, safety, and costs of existing alternatives to the product

- Availability and levels of reimbursement for similar devices

- Reimbursement codes and reimbursement levels for professional and institutional services associated with the product

- Importance of Medicare coverage for the prospective patients.

Almost all interview subjects emphasized early planning of clinical and economic studies. In this regard, subjects suggested that the following steps be taken:

- When planning studies, ask payers what kind of information they would find useful in making coverage and medical-necessity decisions.

- Develop clear, evidence-based guidelines for appropriate use.

- Develop evidence that the FDA does not require for product approval.

- Work with centers of excellence in designing and executing studies.

- Involve in the studies influential physicians who may become champions of the technologies.

- Make sure, however, that those studies that are undertaken are good investments.

PERSPECTIVES OF MCO MEDICAL DIRECTORS

To understand how MCOs respond to the availability of new medical technologies, we sought to interview managed care organizations representing a substantial proportion of the managed care market in California. Each interview addressed five sets of issues:

- The extent of formal technology assessments of new medical devices, the processes employed, and the role of manufacturers

- How the MCO makes coverage decisions for procedures involving emerging medical devices

- How the MCO sets payment or reimbursement levels for medical devices

- How case-by-case medical-necessity determinations are made
- Lessons learned and advice for medical device manufacturers.

All of the interview subjects emphasized that technology adoption for MCOs involves a multilayered process for determining whether a procedure, and any devices involved, will be eligible for payment. Within that process of coverage decisionmaking, formal technology-assessment processes vary widely across MCOs with respect to

- The level of formality, including whether the MCO uses staff in addition to the medical director and one or more standing committees to conduct the technology assessment
- Who is responsible for decisionmaking
- The rigor—depth and breadth—of the review of medical evidence
- The use of outside expertise and resources, including technology-assessment firms and national or local physician experts
- The extent to which MCOs are influenced by governmental organizations and health-insurance-industry leaders
- The average number of formal technology reviews conducted each year.

Technology assessment is usually a closed process, and manufacturers are not allowed to participate directly. Yet MCOs report that they consider information supplied by manufacturers and, while carefully reviewing the design and methodology, accord the same weight to manufacturer-sponsored, peer-reviewed studies as they do to other peer-reviewed studies.

There were varying levels of enthusiasm for joint efforts between manufacturers and MCOs. At least one MCO medical director offered each of the following suggestions:

- Manufacturers should help MCOs anticipate what technologies are "in the pipeline" and the potential costs.
- Manufacturers should share information on experience with medical devices across MCOs and providers.

- Manufacturers and MCOs should foster cooperative research in routine clinical settings.

- Manufacturers and MCOs should facilitate cooperative provider education.

- Manufacturers and MCOs should create contracts that enable the MCOs to upgrade expensive, multi-use devices as improvements are made.

- MCOs should allow manufacturers to participate in technology-assessment processes.

HOW MIGHT TECHNOLOGY ADOPTION BE IMPROVED?

The social goal of adopting or rejecting technologies on the basis of their social costs and benefits involves enormous complexities and uncertainties, and achieving anything close to perfection in winnowing technologies is not possible. However, in view of the size of the U.S. health care system and of the potential contributions of new technology to health, even incremental improvements could have large payoffs.

A major impediment to socially appropriate adoption of emerging medical technologies is limited information about the performance of these technologies—both absolutely and relative to alternative technologies—in day-to-day medical practice. We see prospects for improving four elements of information availability:

- Developing better information before market introduction

- Learning more from experience after market introduction

- Evaluating and synthesizing clinical information

- Disseminating information.

We also discuss several other issues that warrant consideration:

- Aligning private incentives of MCOs and payers with social values

- Enhancing MCO capabilities to evaluate technologies and make decisions

- Improving decisions by physicians
- Reducing use of inappropriate or obsolete technologies
- Reducing costs of decisionmaking for manufacturers and MCOs
- Improving manufacturer understanding of the market environment
- Helping MCOs and employers anticipate what is in the pipeline.

Improving the processes of medical-technology adoption raises numerous, complex issues. The discussion at the October 7 meeting provided reason to hope that representatives of the managed-care and medical-technology industries could engage in constructive, joint exploration of what might be accomplished by private, voluntary action. It was also agreed that it would be very helpful to include payers (e.g., consortia of employers) in such a process. Various issues raised above provide potential agenda items for such discussions.

ACKNOWLEDGMENTS

The research reported here was sponsored by the Health Industry Manufacturers Association (HIMA) with funds provided by the Goldstrike Partnership—a program of the California Trade and Commerce Agency's Office of Strategic Technology—and the Economic Development Administration (EDA) of the U.S. Department of Commerce. We are indebted to several individuals associated with these organizations for aiding our efforts in various ways. Specifically, we thank Pam Bailey (HIMA), Alex Glass (Bay Area Regional Technology Alliance), Maxene Johnston (Johnston and Company), Candace Littell (C.L. & Associates), Jeff Newman (Office of Strategic Technology, California Trade and Commerce Agency), Dee Simons (HIMA), Leonard Smith (EDA), and Deena Sosson (EDA).

We are also indebted to dozens of people who generously provided information that represents the core data used in our analysis. They include individuals at eight companies that manufacture medical devices and nine managed care organizations (MCOs) who participated in confidential interviews and several representatives of manufacturers and MCOs who participated in a meeting held at RAND on October 7, 1999, during which our preliminary findings were critiqued and discussed and additional information was collected. Owing to our pledges of confidentiality, we cannot thank these individuals by name.

We also thank Meg Bernhardt and Dotty Marsh of RAND for helping to arrange interviews and the October 7 meeting. RAND colleagues Rebecca D'Amato and Elizabeth Rolph generously shared notes on literature concerning coverage decisionmaking by health plans. We are grateful to Marian Branch of RAND for excellent and timely editorial assistance. Finally, we thank our technical reviewers— Katherine Harris of RAND and Scott D. Ramsey of the University of Washington—for timely, thoughtful, and constructive comments and suggestions.